The Nordic Cookbook

Delicious Recipes for a Healthy Lifestyle

Author

Elvira P. Cazares

By Elvira P. Cazares, Copyright 2021

The right to use this information is reserved. With the exception of brief excerpts in critical reviews, no part of this book may be reproduced in any form without the publisher's express permission.

Contents

5 1. Ballyvolane Gravadlax with Cucumber Pickle and Dill Mustard Mayonnaise (NORDIC DIET 4 HEALTHY HOMEMADE NORDIC DIET RECIPES)

2. Salad with Shaved Winter Vegetables

Cardamom Buns (number 8)

10 4. Cranberry Sauce with Scandinavian Rice
Pudding

Lohikeitto is a traditional Finnish salmon soup.

19 7. Midsummer Cocktail 21 8. Nordic Open
Faced Smoked Salmon Sandwiches 22 9.
Chewy Apricot Energy Balls 17 6. Icelandic
Pancakes (Pönnukökur) 19 7. Midsummer
Cocktail

25. Almond-Berry French Toast Bake 27. Chipotle Chicken Fajitas 29. Roasted Shrimp Parmesan 31. Curried White Bean Dip 33.

37. Green Bean Casserole with Cashew Cream (Vegan/Dairy Free) 35 15. Roasted Butternut Squash with Frizzled Sage

39 17. Vegetarian Mushroom Gravy 42 18. Pumpkin-Carrot Soup 46 20. Cranberry and Apricot Compote 48 21. Roasted Butternut Squash with Frizzled Sage 50 22. Green Beans with Almond Gremolata 52 23. Herb Smashed Root Veggies 54 24. Beet, Mushroom, and

Avocado Salad 56 25. Vegan Caesar Salad 58 26. Wild Rice-Stuffed Acorn Squash 62 27.

DIET NORWAY

It may surprise you, but meatballs and Danish butter cookies aren't the only foods served in Scandinavia. In fact, eating whole and plant-based foods is a centuries-old tradition in the region that includes Norway, Sweden, Finland, Denmark, and Iceland.

A modern eating style based on these traditional foods is known as the Nordic or Scandinavian diet. Processed foods, sugar, and red meat are limited in the diet, which is high in complex carbohydrates, lean proteins, and healthy fats. It also emphasizes the importance of eating foods that have a lower environmental impact.

RECIPE FOR A HEALTHY NORDIC DIET MADE AT HOME

1. Ballyvolane Gravadlax with Dill Mustard Mayonnaise and Cucumber Pickle

30 minutes in total Servings:8

Ingredients

Gravadlax (salmon)

2 tbsp sea salt, 2 tbsp sugar, 2 tbsp ground black pepper, 4 tbsp chopped fresh dill • 2 tbsp sea salt, 2 tbsp sugar, 2 tbsp ground black pepper To make the Cucumber Pickle, combine the cucumbers, salt, and vinegar in a mixing bowl

1 cucumber • 4 tbsp rice vinegar • 4 tbsp caster sugar • 1 tbsp salt

• 1 very thinly sliced small shallot

• 3 tablespoons boiling water

To make the Dill Mustard Mayonnaise, combine all of the ingredients in a mixing bowl and whisk together until smooth.

1 large egg yolk • 2 tbsp French mustard • 1 tbsp white sugar • 1/2 pint sunflower oil • 1 tbsp white wine vinegar Gravadlax Recipe Instructions:

1. In a large mixing bowl, combine the salt, sugar, pepper, and dill. Spread the mixture evenly over one side of the salmon on cling film.

2. Place the other half of the salmon on top of the prepared side. Refrigerate the salmon completely wrapped in cling film. For four

days, turn this every day. On the fifth day, it will be completed.

To make the Cucumber Pickle, combine the cucumbers, salt, and vinegar in a mixing bowl

1. Slice the cucumber lengthwise in half. If you have a mandolin, slice very thinly.

2. In a mixing bowl, combine the sugar, salt, vinegar, and hot water, then add the cucumber, shallot, and red chilli. Before serving, divide the mixture among individual serving jars and chill overnight.

To make the Dill Mustard Mayonnaise, combine all of the ingredients in a mixing bowl and whisk together until smooth.

1. In a mixing bowl, slowly combine the yolk, mustard, and sugar.

2. Slowly drizzle in the oil until it emulsifies, then whisk in the vinegar and dill. Using salt and pepper, season to taste.

2. Winter Vegetable Salad with Shaved Vegetables

Ingredient

• 4 small radishes • 1 small golden beet • 1 small red beet • 1 black radish • 1 watermelon radish

• olive oil • balsamic glaze or pomegranate molasses • salt and fresh cracked black pepper to taste

Directions

1. Scrub but do not peel the beets and large radishes. Remove the leafy stem end and slice on your mandolin's 1/8 inch setting.

2. Getting the slices just right might require some trial and error. You'd like them to be slim and attractive.

Transparent in appearance. While you're working, place the slices on a damp plate and cover with a damp kitchen towel.

3. Peel and slice the carrots in the same fashion.

4. When doing this, be extremely cautious of your fingers. When possible, use the mandolin's built-in safety guard.

5. Place a layer of dill or a leaf or two of lettuce on each of four small plates to assemble your salads.

6. Begin layering the vegetables in a loose stack with the largest rounds. The smaller carrots should be placed on top.

7. Finish with a balsamic glaze and a drizzle of olive oil. Serve immediately after lightly seasoning with salt and pepper.

Cardamom Buns are the third item on the list.

30 minutes to prepare 15-minutes to cook

Servings:16

2 cups plus 2 tablespoons whole milk • 1/2 cup plus 2 tablespoons unsalted butter

• 2 packages instant yeast (each package contains 1/2 oz. of yeast, or 4 1/2 teaspoons.)

For the filling, combine 1 teaspoon salt, 1/2 cup granulated sugar, and 5 3/4 cups all-purpose flour.

For the glaze, combine 10 tablespoons unsalted butter, 1/2 cup granulated sugar, and 1 1/2 teaspoons ground cardamom

• 1/4 cup water • 1/2 teaspoon vanilla extract

Directions

1. Melt the butter in a small saucepan, followed by the milk.

2. In the bowl of a stand mixer fitted with the dough hook attachment, warm the mixture until it is lukewarm.

3. Combine the yeast, milk, and butter in a mixing bowl and stir to combine. After that, combine the salt and sugar.

4. Slowly drizzle in the flour while the mixer is on low speed. Continue kneading for about 10 minutes after all of the flour has been added.

5. The dough should be smooth and begin to pull away from the bowl's side.

6. Allow to rise for 45 minutes to an hour, or until nearly doubled in size (no need to transfer to a separate greased bowl).

7. Make the cardamom filling while the dough is rising by mixing all of the filling ingredients together with a fork until uniform. It's best if your butter is soft enough to easily mix. Remove the item from circulation.

8. Line two large baking sheets with parchment paper to prevent them from sticking together.

9. Gently deflate and divide the dough after it has risen. Roll out one half of the dough into a 14-inch-wide by 18-inch-long rectangle on a lightly floured surface. Half of the filling should be spread out over half of the rolled out rectangle.

10. Fold the half of the dough that hasn't been filled over the other half. Roll out the dough a little more to get a fairly even thickness across the board.

11. Cut your folded rectangle into 8 equal strips widthwise using a knife or a pizza cutter.

12. Cut each strip in half lengthwise, leaving a small gap at the top.

13. Gently twist each "leg" in the same direction as the others.

After that, gently twist the two "legs" together.

15. To keep your twist from unraveling, coil it into a small circle, tucking the end underneath and pinching it into place. Don't worry about being perfect; just twist everything into a'messy bun.'

16. Continue with the other half of the dough and the remaining rectangles.

17. Arrange the shaped rolls on the prepared baking sheets, a few inches apart. Allow to rise for about 1 hour before covering loosely with a kitchen towel. They shouldn't puff up as much as they did before, but they should be plumper.

Preheat the oven to 425 degrees Fahrenheit near the end of the rising time.

19. Bake for 15 minutes after the buns have finished rising.

20. To make the glaze, combine the sugar and water in a small saucepan and heat over low heat until the sugar is dissolved.

The sugar has been broken down. Take the pot off the heat and add the vanilla extract.

21. Remove the buns from the oven when they're done baking and glaze them while they're still warm. If you want them to be

extra-shiny, you can apply a second coat of glaze after they've cooled down.

4. Cranberry Sauce and Scandinavian Rice Pudding

45 minutes to prepare 45 minutes in total

Servings:6

Ingredients

• 5 cups whole milk • 1 cup cream • 1 heaping cup arborio rice • 2/3 cup granulated sugar •

1/2 teaspoon ground cardamom • vanilla bean seeds • cranberry sauce

• 3 cups cranberries in their natural state • 1/2 cup sugar • a splash of water

Directions

2. Bring the milk, cream, rice, sugar, cardamom, and vanilla seeds to a boil in a saucepan.

3. Reduce the heat to low and cook for 40-45 minutes, uncovered, until the sauce has

thickened. Stir frequently, and after about 30 minutes, when it begins to thicken, pay closer attention.

4. Make sure it doesn't burn on the pan's bottom or sides. When the rice is plump and tender and the custard has thickened slightly, the pudding is ready to serve. It's worth noting that as the rice pudding cools, it will thicken even more.

5. Spoon the pudding into small bowls or glasses for serving. Allow to cool before chilling until ready to use. If you prefer, you can serve it hot. Serve cranberry sauce on the side.

6. To make the cranberry sauce, in a saucepan, combine the cranberries, sugar, and a splash of

water and bring to a simmer, stirring constantly to dissolve the sugar.

7. Cook, stirring frequently, until the berries burst and the sauce is glossy, about 5 minutes. On top of the pudding, this can be served warm or chilled.

5. Lohikeitto – a traditional Finnish salmon soup

10 Minutes to Prepare 20 minutes to prepare 30 minutes total time Servings:4

Ingredient

1 pound skin-on salmon filet • 4 tablespoons unsalted butter • 1 large leek, trimmed, sliced, and well rinsed • 5 cups water (you can also use fish stock) • 1 pound russet potatoes, peeled and diced • 1 large carrot, sliced • 1 cup fresh dill for garnish, finely chopped, divided

Directions

1. Cut the salmon into large chunks after removing the skin. Small pin bones should be removed and thrown away. The skin should be kept separate.

2. In a soup pot, melt the butter and cook the leeks for 10 minutes, or until soft.

3. While the leeks are cooking, in a saucepan, bring 5 cups of water and the reserved fish skin to a boil, then reduce to a low heat and allow to simmer for 10 minutes. This step can be skipped if using fish stock.

4. Strain the broth and add the potatoes, carrots, and half of the fresh dill to the pan with the leeks. Cook for an additional 10 minutes, or until the potatoes are barely tender.

5. Add the salmon chunks, cream, and allspice to the soup and gently simmer for a few minutes, or until cooked through. Season with salt and pepper and the remaining dill.

7. Pönnukökur (Icelandic Pancakes)

5 Minutes Preparation 10 minutes to prepare

15 minutes in total

Ingredient

• 2 c flour • 1 tbsp sugar • 18 tsp baking soda •

2 eggs • 1-2 tsp cardamom (or vanilla) (melted)

• as needed, milk

Directions

In a mixing bowl, combine the dry ingredients.

2. melted butter, and vanilla extract in a

separate mixing bowl

3. Combine the ingredients in a slow, steady

stream to form a thin, smooth batter.

After that, slowly pour in the milk.

, and whisk until a runny batter is formed.

4. Allow 30 minutes for the batter to settle.

5. Melt the butter in a skillet over medium heat

until fragrant; pour in enough batter to thinly

coat the skillet (pancakes should be very thin).

Cook until the bottom of the thin pancake is

lightly browned, then flip to brown the other side.

6. Be sure to rotate the pan after pouring the batter into it. This makes it easier for the batter to spread thinly and quickly across the baking sheet.

7. Toss it on a plate with cinnamon and sugar and roll it up tightly, or stack it on a plate to fold in whipped cream and preserves or fruit once it's done.

Cocktail for the Midsummer

Ingredient

• 1 1/2 oz aquavit • 3/4 oz sherry manzanilla •

1/4 oz St. Germain elderflower liqueur

• garnish with a twist of lemon (optional)

Directions

1. In a mixing glass full of ice, combine all of
your ingredients and stir for 30 to 40 seconds.

2. Strain into a chilled coupe glass with a
lemon twist as a garnish.

8. Smoked Salmon Sandwiches in a Nordic Style

15 minutes to prepare 5 minutes to prepare

Ingredient

• butter at room temperature • homemade dilled mayonnaise recipe below • salt and freshly cracked black pepper • thin slices of smoked salmon • microgreens • edible flowers

• dilled mayonnaise • lemon as a garnish

1 room-temperature pasteurized egg

• 1 cup room temperature olive oil with a mild flavor

• a handful of fresh dill • seasoning to taste with salt and pepper • a squeeze of lemon

Direcions

Preheat the oven to 400 degrees Fahrenheit (200 degrees Celsius).

2. Make smaller rectangles out of the bread slices. If you prefer, you can make them smaller. Spread a thin layer of soft butter on each slice and toast in the oven for a few minutes, or until they begin to crisp up.

3. You can use the bread without being toasted if you prefer.

4. Spread a thin layer of dilled mayonnaise on each slice of bread, then top with smoked salmon slices.

5. Toss in the microgreens, season with salt and pepper, and serve. Serve with small lemon wedges and an edible flower as a finishing touch.

6. To make homemade mayonnaise, combine the room temperature egg, oil, and dill in a jar large enough to fit an immersion blender.

7. Place the blender in the bottom of the jar and turn it on, gradually elevating the blade as the mixture is emulsified. It will just take 30 seconds to complete this task. Stop cooking until the sauce has turned into mayonnaise.

blending. The salt and pepper, as well as a little lemon juice, may be added at this point.

9. Apricot Energy Balls that are chewy and delicious

15 minutes in total Servings:10

Ingredient

• 1/2 cup blanched slivered almonds • 1 cup dried apricots • 2 tablespoons unsweetened shredded coconut • 1 tablespoon white chia seeds • 1 tablespoon honey • 1/2 teaspoon pure vanilla essence • 1/8 teaspoon crushed cardamom • 1/8 teaspoon kosher salt • shredded coconut

Directions

1. Pulse slivered almonds in a food processor until finely chopped. Process to finely chop the dried apricots, shredded coconut, chia seeds, honey, vanilla essence, powdered cardamom, and kosher salt.

2. Make 1-inch balls with the mixture (about 1 heaping tbsp. each). Roll in coconut flakes if desired. Keep refrigerated for up to one week in an airtight container.

10. Baked French Toast with Almonds and Berries Total Time: 4 Hours Servings:9

Ingredient

6 to 8 oz. raspberries • 6 big eggs • 2 large egg whites • 2 1/4 c. 2 percent milk • 3 tbsp. pure maple syrup • 2 tsp. pure vanilla extract • 3/4 tsp. crushed cinnamon • 1/2 tsp. kosher salt •

1/4 c. old-fashioned oats • 1/4 c. chopped almonds

Directions

1. Using cooking spray, lightly coat a shallow 1 1/2-quart baking dish. Evenly distribute the bread pieces and raspberries.

2. Whisk eggs, egg whites, milk, maple syrup, vanilla, cinnamon, and salt together in a large mixing dish. Cover and chill for 3 hours.

3. Preheat the oven to 350 degrees Fahrenheit (180 degrees Celsius). Top with oats and

almonds and bake for 40 to 50 minutes, or until puffed and golden brown.

Chicken Fajitas with Chipotle Sauce

30 minutes in total Servings:4

Ingredients

1 pound boneless, skinless chicken breasts, thinly sliced • 1 teaspoon ground cumin • 1 teaspoon chili powder • kosher salt • pepper

• 1 tablespoon canola oil • 1 red pepper, sliced

• 1 small onion, sliced • 1 cup sliced mushrooms • 3 garlic cloves, minced • 1 tablespoon chopped chipotle chiles in adobo chiles in adobo chiles in adobo chiles in adobo chiles in adobo chiles in adobo chiles in adobo chiles in adobo

• serving lime wedges Directions

1. Season the chicken with cumin, chili powder, and a quarter teaspoon of salt and pepper.

2. In a large cast-iron skillet, heat the oil to a high temperature. Cook, tossing regularly, for 5 to 7 minutes, or until the chicken is cooked through. Place on a platter and serve.

3. Add red pepper, onion, mushrooms, and garlic to the same skillet and cook, stirring periodically, for 4 to 6 minutes, or until tender.

4. Add the chipotle peppers, lime juice, and chicken, as well as a sprinkle of salt and pepper. Stir constantly until the mixture is thoroughly hot.

5. Arrange chicken and veggies on tortillas with desired toppings.

12. Shrimp Parmesan with Roasted Garlic

40 minutes in total Servings:4

Ingredient

- 6 oz. rustic bread, broken into 3/4-inch pieces

- kosher salt • pepper • 3 tablespoons olive oil, divided

1 pound plum tomatoes, sliced into 1/2-inch chunks • 2 garlic cloves, coarsely chopped

- 1 tiny basil bunch, torn and separated leaves

- 1 pound big peeled and deveined shrimp • 3 ounces shredded mozzarella cheese (about 1 cup) • 3 tablespoons grated Parmesan cheese

Directions

Preheat the oven to 425 degrees Fahrenheit (200 degrees Celsius). In a large oven-safe skillet, heat 2 tablespoons oil on low heat.

2. Toss the bread in the oil to coat it, then season with 1/4 teaspoon salt and 1/4 teaspoon pepper.

3. Bake in the oven for 8 to 10 minutes, or until the bread is golden brown and crunchy.

4. Remove the bread from the pan and add the remaining tbsp. oil and garlic.

5. Cook, stirring occasionally, for approximately 1 minute, or until the garlic becomes golden brown.

6. Add the tomatoes and 1/4 teaspoon each of salt and pepper, and simmer, stirring periodically, for 5 to 7 minutes, or until the

tomatoes start to release their juices. Half of the basil leaves should be folded in at this point.

7. In a large mixing bowl, combine the shrimp and bread. Bake for 14 to 16 minutes, or until the shrimp are opaque and the cheese is golden brown and bubbling. Serve right away with the rest of the basil on top.

13. White Bean Dip with Curried Curried Curried Curried Curried Curried White Bean

10 minutes in total Servings:4

Ingredient

• 2 tbsp olive oil, with a little more for serving

2 tsp. curry powder • 1 big garlic clove, squeezed

• 1 tbsp. fresh lemon juice • 1 15-oz. container drained white beans

For serving, combine kosher salt, pepper, and cilantro.

• pita bread (to serve) that has been toasted

• serving cucumbers • serving peppers

Directions

1. Heat the oil, garlic, curry powder, and 1 teaspoon grated lemon zest in a small pan until the garlic is fragrant, approximately 2 minutes.

2. Puree white beans, lemon juice, salt, and pepper until smooth in a tiny food processor.

3. Transfer to a bowl and top with cilantro and more oil. For dipping, provide toasted pita, cucumbers, and peppers.

14. Kale-Smothered Roasted Chicken & Potatoes

40 minutes in total Servings:4

Ingredients

- 1 pound yellow potatoes, sliced into 3/4-inch chunks • 1/2 cup green olives • 2 teaspoons fresh thyme leaves

- black pepper • kosher salt

1 tsp. paprika 1 lemon, halved

- 4 small chicken legs, cut in half (4 drumsticks and 4 thighs; 2 1/2 lbs.)

- baby kale, 4 c.

Directions

Preheat the oven to 425 degrees Fahrenheit (200 degrees Celsius). Toss potatoes, olives, and thyme with 2 tbsp. on a large rimmed baking sheet.

2 tbsp. oil, 1/4 tbsp. salt, and 1/4 tbsp. pepper Cut sides down, place lemon halves on baking sheet.

3. Combine paprika, the remaining tbsp. oil, and 1/2 tsp. salt and pepper in a small mixing dish.

4. Rub the chicken with the mixture and place it on a baking sheet amid the veggies.

5. Roast chicken and veggies for 25 to 30 minutes, or until golden brown and well cooked.

6. Remove the chicken to plates, spread the kale over the vegetables in the pan, and return to the oven for 1 minute, or until the kale is just starting to wilt. Combine kale and potatoes in a mixing bowl, then drizzle with lemon juice and serve with chicken.

15. Frizzled Sage with Roasted Butternut Squash

15-Minute Prep 30 minutes in total Servings:8

Ingredients

• 2 small butternut squash • 1/3 cup olive oil, plus enough for the baking pan • 1/3 cup fresh sage leaves (each about 2 lbs)

• salt and pepper (Kosher)

Directions

Preheat the oven to 400 degrees Fahrenheit (200 degrees Celsius). Oil the foil and line a rimmed baking sheet.

2. In a small saucepan, heat the oil over medium-high heat. Cook, stirring constantly,

for 1 minute, or until the sage leaves are crisp. Reserve the oil and place the leaves on a paper towel–lined dish.

3. Cut the butternut squash in half lengthwise and remove the seeds. Using a pointed object

Using a paring knife, crisscross the squash's neck flesh.

4. Season squash with 34 tsp salt and 14 tsp pepper while working on the prepared baking sheet with 2 tbsp sage oil.

5. Roast the squash cut side down in the lowest part of the oven for 30 to 35 minutes, or until the flesh starts to become golden brown. Roast

for another 45 to 55 minutes, or until the squash skin is golden brown and crunchy. 6. sage leaves, crispy

16. (Vegan/Dairy-Free) Green Bean Casserole with Cashew Cream

25 minutes to prepare 50 minutes in total

Servings:8

Ingredients

• 2 cups vegetable broth (if not vegan, replace with chicken or turkey broth/stock)

1 pound cremini (baby bella) mushrooms • 1 cup finely chopped yellow onion (sub shallots) • 1 Tbsp. sherry vinegar • 3 garlic cloves, minced • 2 tsp. fresh thyme leaves • 3/4 tsp. kosher salt, divided • 1/2 tsp. black pepper • 1/4 tsp. powdered nutmeg • 1 pound fresh green beans, snapped in half

• 5 ounces sourdough bread, broken into tiny pieces (ideally 1 day old)

Directions

1. In a small saucepan, combine the broth and bay leaves; heat to a boil over high heat.

2. When the water has reached a boil, add the cashews and turn off the heat. While you finish the rest of the dish, soak the cashews in the boiling broth.

Preheat the oven to 425 degrees Fahrenheit.

4. In a large pan over medium-high heat, heat 2 tablespoons of oil.

5. When the pan is heated, add the mushrooms and onion and cook, turning periodically, for 10 to 12 minutes, or until tender. Combine the vinegar, garlic, thyme, 1/2 teaspoon salt, and black pepper in a large mixing bowl. Cook for 3 to 5 minutes, or until the vinegar smell has

faded and the garlic has developed a pleasant perfume. Heat should be turned off.

6. Discard bay leaves and puree cashews and broth in a high-powered blender.

7. Blend in the remaining 1/4 teaspoon salt for approximately 60 seconds, or until the mixture is smooth.

a creamy and silky texture (it should resemble milk). Pour the mixture into the mushroom pan with care. Stir in the nutmeg well.

8. Use nonstick cooking spray to grease an 11x7-inch baking dish. Pour the cashew

mushroom cream mixture over the green beans in the pan. Toss with a pair of tongs.

9. Toss the torn sourdough with the remaining 2 tablespoons olive oil and a sprinkle of salt in a large mixing dish. Toss the bread with the oil in your hands, carefully kneading it into the crevices. Transfer the skillet to the oven with the bread strewn over the green bean casserole. Bake for 20 to 25 minutes, uncovered, or until the sourdough is golden brown and the dish is bubbling. Before serving, set aside for 5 to 10 minutes.

17. Mushroom Gravy with Vegetarian Options

10 minutes to prepare 15 minutes in total

Servings:8

Ingredients

• kosher salt • 2 tbsp extra-virgin olive oil • 1/2 onion, finely chopped • 4 oz. mushrooms, coarsely chopped

• 3 tbsp all-purpose flour • 3 c vegetable stock • 1 tsp chopped thyme • 1 tsp chopped sage • 1 tsp chopped rosemary

Directions

1. In a small saucepan, heat the olive oil on medium. Sauté the onion for 6 minutes, or until tender.

Season with salt and pepper after the mushrooms and herbs have been added. Cook for another 5 minutes until the vegetables are tender. Cook 1 minute after adding the flour.

2. Whisk together 2 cups vegetable stock. Cook, stirring occasionally, for 5-10 minutes, until the flavors have merged and the sauce has thickened somewhat. If the sauce becomes too thick, add additional vegetable stock gradually.

3. Season with extra salt and pepper to taste, if necessary, and serve warm.

Salad with Pumpkin Seed Oil and Roasted Pumpkin and Pomegranates Vinaigrette

45 minutes in total Servings:4

Ingredient

• 6 c. mixed winter salad greens • 1/2 c. pomegranate seeds • 8 tsp. gently roasted pumpkin seeds • 1/4 c. crumbled goat cheese 3 tbsp pure pumpkin-seed oil (available in health-food shops and specialized markets) • 2

tbsp champagne vinegar • 3 orange juice • 1 tsp

dijon mustard • 1 tiny chopped shallot

Vinaigrette: (makes 1/2 cup) (1 Tbsp)

• 1/4 tsp. salt • 1/4 tsp. pepper • 1 tsp. honey

Directions

Preheat the oven to 400 degrees Fahrenheit

(200 degrees Celsius). Toss the pumpkin with

the olive oil, salt, and pepper, then spread it out

on a lipped baking sheet in a single layer.

2. Roast for approximately 30 minutes, or until the pumpkin is tender-firm and the edges have caramelized. Allow to cool fully after removing from oven.

3. In a small jar with a tight-fitting lid, whisk together all of the vinaigrette ingredients until the dressing emulsifies and becomes creamy.

4. Arrange the greens on four salad dishes in an equitable distribution. On top of each dish of greens, sprinkle 1/2 cup roasted pumpkin, 1 tablespoon pomegranate seeds, 2 tablespoons pumpkin seeds, and 1 tablespoon goat cheese. 2 teaspoons vinaigrette drizzled over salad

Soup made with pumpkin and carrots (nineteenth)

35 minutes to prepare 30 minutes to prepare 1 hour 5 minutes total Servings:4

Ingredient

• 2 3/4 pound sugar pumpkin, peeled and cut 1/2 inch thick (seeds retained) • 1 pound carrots, thinly sliced • 1 onion, finely sliced • 2 garlic cloves, thinly sliced • 2 sprigs fresh sage

Directions

1. In a large saucepan over medium heat, heat 1 tbsp oil. Cook, covered, for 12 minutes, turning occasionally, until pumpkin, carrots, onion, garlic, sage, and 1/2 teaspoon salt and pepper are soft. Cook 1 minute after stirring in the nutmeg.

2. Bring 5 cups water to a boil, then reduce to a low heat and continue to cook for 5 to 7 minutes, or until veggies are soft. Remove the sage leaves and purée the soup in batches using an immersion blender (or a regular blender).

3. Preheat the oven to 400 degrees Fahrenheit while you're waiting. Toss the saved pumpkin seeds with the remaining 2 tablespoons of oil on a rimmed baking sheet.

4. Add the oil, a bit of salt, and a pinch of pepper to the pan and cook, stirring once, for 18 to 20 minutes, or until golden brown and crisp. If preferred, finish with a sprinkle of olive oil and seeds on top of the soup.

Compote de cranberries et d'apricot

40 minutes in total Servings:8

Ingredients

- 1 teaspoon of extra virgin olive oil

• 2 shallots, finely chopped • 8 oz. unsulfured dried apricots, very finely chopped — 1 pound fresh or frozen cranberries • 2 teaspoons fresh thyme leaves, plus extra for serving

Directions

In a medium saucepan, heat the oil and shallots on low heat. Cook for approximately 2 minutes, stirring occasionally, until the vegetables are soft.

2. Bring 112 cup water to a boil with the apricots and 12 teaspoon salt. Reduce to a low

heat and continue to cook, covered, for 8 to 10 minutes, or until softened.

3. Stir in the cranberries and 1 teaspoon thyme and continue to cook, covered, for another 15 to 20 minutes, or until the cranberries have broken down and the sauce has thickened.

4. Add the 14 tsp pepper and the remaining tsp thyme. If preferred, top with more thyme and serve warm or at room temperature.

21. Frizzled Sage and Roasted Butternut Squash

15-Minute Prep 30 minutes in total Servings:8

Ingredients

• 2 small butternut squash • 1/3 cup olive oil,
plus enough for the baking pan • 1/3 cup fresh
sage leaves (each about 2 lbs)

• salt and pepper (Kosher)

Directions

Preheat the oven to 400 degrees Fahrenheit
(200 degrees Celsius). Oil the foil and line a
rimmed baking sheet.

2. In a small saucepan, heat the oil over medium-high heat. Cook, stirring constantly, for 1 minute, or until the sage leaves are crisp.

3. Drain the oil and place the leaves on a paper towel–lined dish.

Scoop out and remove the seeds after cutting butternut squash in half lengthwise.

4. Score the squash neck flesh in a crisscross pattern with a sharp paring knife.

5. Season squash with 34 tsp salt and 14 tsp pepper while working on the prepared baking sheet with 2 tbsp sage oil.

6. Roast the squash cut side down in the lowest part of the oven for 30 to 35 minutes, or until the flesh starts to become golden brown. Roast for another 45 to 55 minutes, or until the squash skin is golden brown and crunchy.

22. Almond Gremolata on Green Beans

15-Minute Prep 5 minutes to cook 20 minutes in total Servings:8

Ingredient

• 1 big onion, finely chopped • 2 tbsp. white wine vinegar • 4 tbsp. olive oil, split • 1 garlic clove, finely minced • 1 tsp. chopped fresh rosemary • 1/2 cup toasted almonds, coarsely chopped — 2 tsp. grated orange zest • 1/2 c. flat-leaf parsley, chopped

Directions

1. Boil a big kettle of water. Toss shallot with vinegar in a large mixing basin and set aside.

2. Heat 2 tablespoons oil, garlic, and rosemary in a small pan over medium heat until garlic sizzles around the edges and becomes brown, approximately 2 minutes. Remove the pan

from the heat and stir in the almonds, zest, and parsley.

3. Add cold water to the bowl. Simmer 1 tbsp. salt in boiling water for 3 minutes, then add half of the green beans and cook until just cooked. Place in cold water using a slotted spoon. Remove and pat dry after it's cooled. Replace the beans and repeat the process.

4. Stir in the remaining 2 tablespoons oil, as well as 1/2 teaspoon salt and pepper, into the shallot mixture. Toss the green beans with the vinaigrette, transfer to a serving tray, and top with the almond mixture.

23. Root Vegetables with Herbs Smashed

20-Minute Prep 25 minutes to prepare 45 minutes in total Servings:8

Ingredient

- 1 pound peeled parsnips • 6 garlic cloves, peeled and coarsely chopped

- 1 pound Yukon gold potatoes, peeled and chopped into 1/2-inch chunks

- 1 pound peeled and sliced carrots

- 6 sprigs fresh thyme • 4 sprigs fresh rosemary

- 4 sprigs fresh flat-leaf parsley

Directions

1. Cut out and remove woody cores from parsnips by quartering them lengthwise. Parsnips should be cut into 1-inch lengths.

2. In a large saucepan, combine the parsnips, garlic, rutabaga, potatoes, carrots, and herbs with cold water and bring to a boil. Simmer, covered, for 12 to 15 minutes, or until veggies are soft.

3. Take the herbs out of the pot and throw them away. Drain and return the veggies to the saucepan with 1/2 cup of the cooking liquid. Drizzle olive oil over the vegetables and season with 1/2 teaspoon of salt and pepper.

4. season to taste with salt and pepper, and mash the veggies using a potato masher (adding some of the reserved liquid if vegetables seem dry). If preferred, serve with chives on top.

Salad with beets, mushrooms, and avocado (number 24)

10 Minutes to Prepare 20 minutes to cook 30 minutes in total Servings:4

Ingredient

4 medium portobello mushroom caps • 1/4 cup lemon juice • 3 tablespoons olive oil • 1 small onion, finely chopped • 5 ounces baby kale • 8 ounces precooked beets, diced • 2 ripe avocados, thinly sliced

Directions

1. Coat portobello mushroom caps with nonstick cooking spray and place on a wide rimmed baking sheet.

Roast for 20 minutes at 450°F or until tender, sprinkled with 1/2 teaspoon salt.

2. Toss half of the dressing with young kale and beets, whisking together the lemon juice, olive oil, shallot, and 1/4 teaspoon salt and pepper. Distribute the mixture among the plates.

3. Add thinly sliced portobellos, avocados, and matzo to the top. On the side, serve the leftover dressing.

Salad Caesar (vegan) No. 25

1 HOUR 45 MINUTES TOTAL Servings:4

Ingredient

To make Crispy Chickpeas, combine all ingredients in a large mixing bowl and mix well.

- 1 can chickpeas (15 oz.) • 1 tablespoon olive oil • Kosher salt and pepper

- 1/4 cup olive oil • 1 tsp. grated lemon zest + 1/3 cup lemon juice • 1/4 cup tahini • 1 tbsp. nutritional yeast • 1 tbsp. Dijon mustard

- 1 small garlic clove, coarsely grated • Kosher salt and pepper

Salad dressings

2 bunches of radishes • 4 thick slices bread • 3
tablespoons olive oil • 2 small red onions,
sliced into thick rounds • Kosher salt and
pepper

• 2 heads gem lettuce or romaine hearts,
separated leaves • 1 garlic clove, split in half

Directions

To make the Crispy Chickpeas, begin by combining all of the ingredients in a large mixing bowl.

Preheat the oven to 425 degrees Fahrenheit (200 degrees Celsius). Rinse chickpeas thoroughly and pat dry with paper towels, discarding any loose skins.

2. Toss chickpeas with 1/4 teaspoon each of salt and pepper on a rimmed baking sheet. Cook for 30 to 40 minutes, shaking occasionally.

3. Transfer to a bowl and toss with lemon zest after removing from the oven. As the chickpeas cool, they will become crisper.

To make the salad and the dressing, start by combining all of the ingredients in a mixing bowl.

1. Preheat the grill to medium-high temperature. To make the dressing, combine all dressing ingredients in a mini blender or food processor and puree until smooth, adding 1 tablespoon water at a time to adjust consistency and seasoning to taste. Discard the dressing.

2. To make the salad, brush 1 1/2 tablespoons of oil on the bread slices. 1 tablespoon oil, 1/4

teaspoon salt and 1/4 teaspoon pepper, brushed on onion slices

3. Season radishes with a pinch of salt and the remaining 1/2 tablespoon oil. On small skewers, thread radishes. 2 to 3 minutes per side on the grill, until toasty; rub with garlic immediately. Onions and radishes should be grilled until tender, about 5 minutes per side for onions and 6 to 8 minutes for radishes.

4. Separate onion rings and tear bread into pieces. Toss half of the dressing with the lettuce to evenly coat it.

Fold in the onion rings and grilled croutons gently. Serve alongside radish skewers, crispy chickpeas, and any leftover dressing for drizzling or dipping.

Prep Time: 20 minutes 26. Wild Rice-Stuffed Acorn Squash 20 minutes to cook 40 minutes in total Servings:8

Ingredient

• 1 cup wild and brown rice blend • 1 bunch spinach, thick stems discarded, leaves roughly chopped • 4 small acorn squash (approximately 4 1/2 pounds total) • 3 tablespoons olive oil

• black pepper • kosher salt

• 1 large onion, finely chopped • 2 garlic cloves, pressed • 2 tsp. fresh thyme leaves

Directions

1. Preheat oven to 425°F and place rimmed baking sheet in it. Cook the rice as directed on the package. Remove pot from heat, top with spinach, cover with clean dishtowel and lid, and set aside for 5 minutes.

2. Cut 1/2 inch off each pointy end of the squash, then half it through the center (this will help it stand straight); spoon out and discard seeds. 1 tbsp oil, 1/4 tsp salt, 1/4 tsp pepper,

squash Roast until tender, 25 to 30 minutes, on a baking sheet with hollow sides down.

3. Meanwhile, in a large skillet over medium heat the remaining 2 tbsp oil. Cook, covered, for 8 minutes, stirring occasionally, with 1/2 teaspoon salt and 1/4 teaspoon pepper.

4. Remove the lid and continue to cook, stirring occasionally, for another 6 to 8 minutes, or until the onion is very tender and golden brown. Remove from heat after 2 minutes of stirring in garlic and thyme.

5. Place squash hollow sides up on a serving platter. Along with the onion, mix in the spinach and scallions.

mixture, then spoon into squash halves. If desired, garnish with more scallions.

27. Pear, Sweet Potato, and Onion Roasted

55 minutes in total Servings:8

Ingredient

• 2 cored and cut into wedges Bartlett pears (approximately 14 oz)

• 2 wedges of small red onions

• 2 small sweet potatoes (about 1 pound), cut into 1/2-inch-thick half-moons • 6 sprigs thyme, plus more for serving

Directions

Preheat the oven to 425 degrees Fahrenheit (200 degrees Celsius). Toss pears, onions, sweet potatoes, and thyme with 1 teaspoon each of salt and pepper on a large rimmed baking sheet.

2. Roast for 35 to 45 minutes, or until golden and tender.

3. If desired, garnish with more thyme.

28. 5 Minute Fresh Cranberry Relish 5 minutes
in total

Ingredient

- 1 pound cranberries • 1 cup granulated sugar

- 1 orange's juice and zest, plus additional

servings (optional)

- kosher salt, 3/4 teaspoon

- 1 tsp cinnamon (ground)

Directions

1. In a food processor, pulse all of the ingredients until the berries are broken down.

2. Store in the refrigerator until ready to eat. If desired, top with additional zest.

29. Vegan Nacho Sauce with Crispy Potatoes

Ingredient

• 2 lb. halved mixed baby potatoes • 3 tbsp. canola oil • 1 c. unsalted raw cashews, soaked overnight and drained • 3 tbsp. lemon juice •

1/2 tsp. chili powder • 1/2 tsp. ground cumin •

1/2 tsp. sweet paprika • 1/2 tsp. garlic powder •

1 tsp. coarse sea salt

Directions

Preheat the oven to 450 degrees Fahrenheit

(230 degrees Celsius). Combine the potatoes,

oil, 1/2 teaspoon salt, and 1/4 teaspoon pepper

in a large mixing bowl. Spread potatoes out

evenly on a rimmed baking sheet; roast for 30

minutes, stirring once, until golden and crisp.

2. Puree the cashews, lemon juice, chili powder, cumin, paprika, garlic powder, sea salt, nutritional yeast, and jalapeno in a blender with 1 cup water until smooth. Heat on medium-low for 5 minutes or until warm, stirring occasionally, in a 2-quart saucepan. 1 2/3 cup (approximately) Serve with roasted potatoes in a mixing bowl. (The remaining sauce can be refrigerated for up to 1 day.) Also delicious with tortilla chips, roasted cauliflower, and other similar dishes.)

Brussels Sprouts with Mustard Glaze

25 minutes in total Servings:8

Ingredient

• 2 pound small Brussels sprouts, trimmed and halved lengthwise • kosher salt • pepper • 4 tablespoons olive oil, divided

• 1/4 cup apricot jam • 3 tablespoons white wine vinegar • 1 tablespoon whole-grain mustard • pinch red pepper flakes (optional) • 4 garlic cloves thinly sliced

Directions

In a large skillet, bring 1/2 cup water and 2 tablespoons oil to a boil. Season with salt and pepper.

Cook, covered, for 5 minutes, stirring occasionally, with 1/2 teaspoon salt.

2. Meanwhile, combine jam, vinegar, mustard, 1/2 teaspoon cracked black pepper, and red pepper flakes, if using, in a small mixing bowl.

3. Remove the lid from the skillet, increase the heat to medium-high, and cook for 2 minutes, or until all of the liquid has evaporated. Cook, tossing occasionally, until Brussels sprouts are golden brown and tender, 2 to 3 minutes.

4. Toss the pepitas with the jam mixture and

cook for 1 minute.

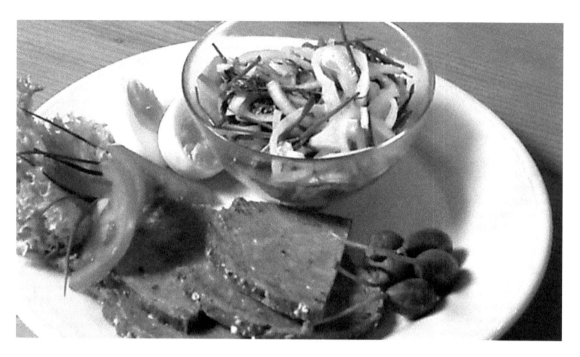
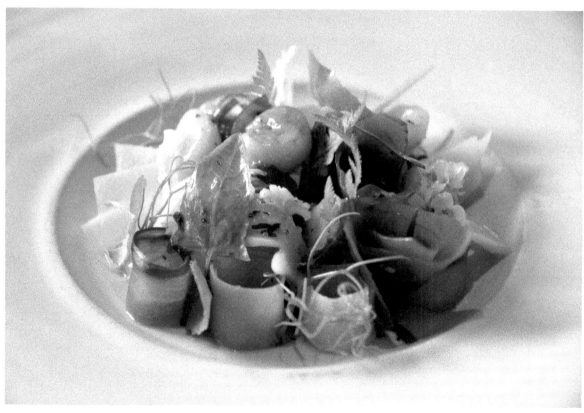

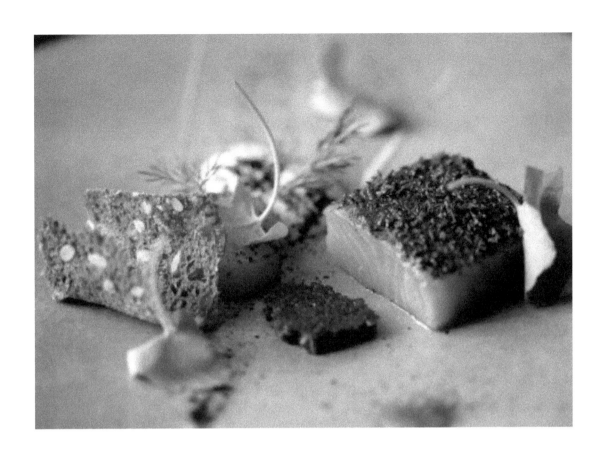

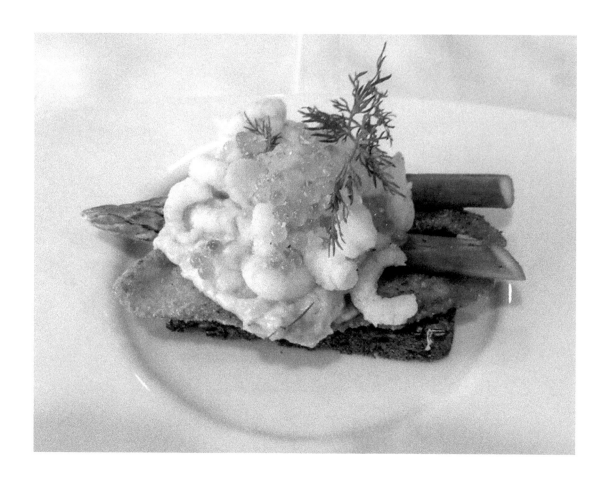

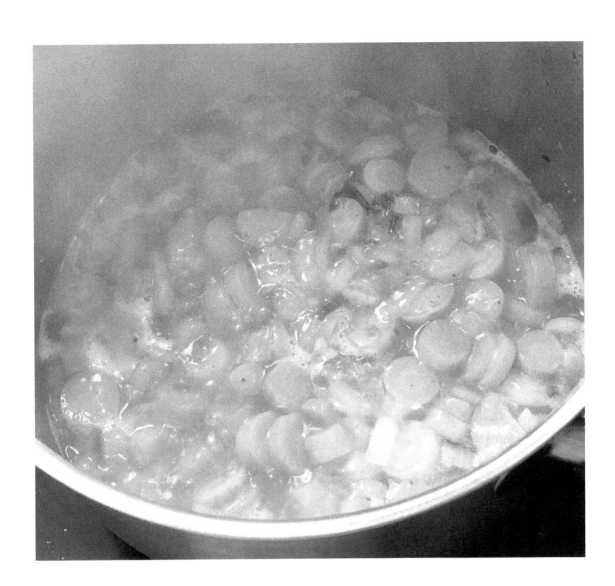

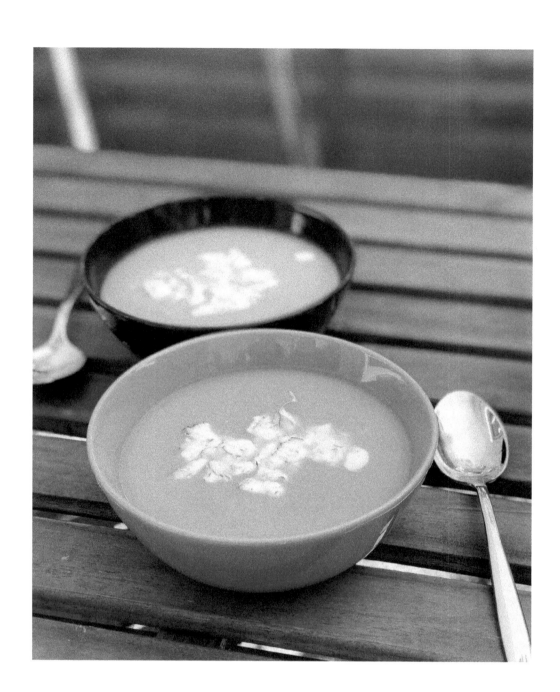

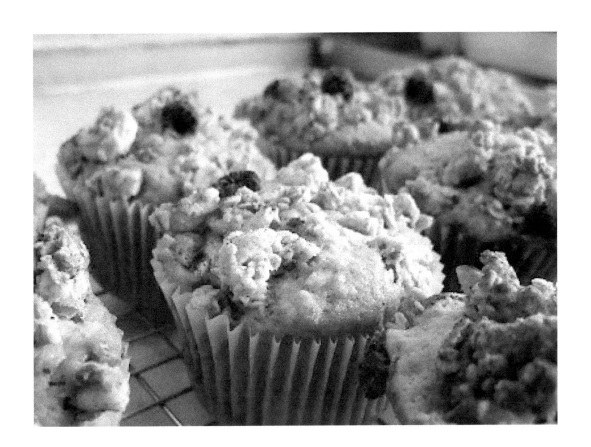

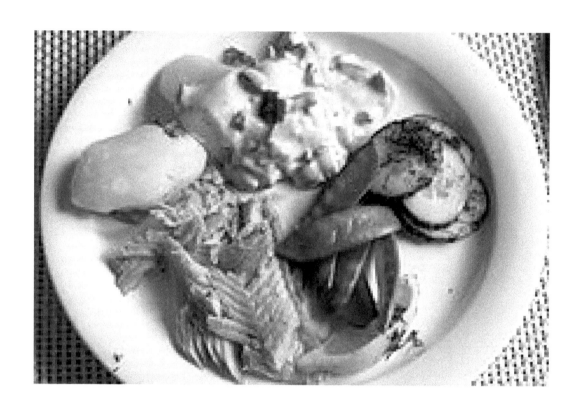

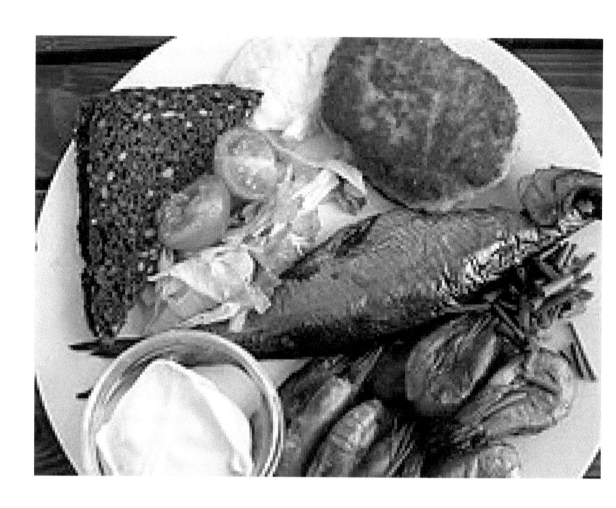

CPSIA information can be obtained
at www.ICGtesting.com
Printed in the USA
LVHW060746221221
706918LV00008B/381